Copyright

© 2023 by Henry H. Welch

Disclaimer

The information provided in this book is for general informational purposes only. The author and publisher make no representations or warranties about the accuracy, completeness, or suitability of the information contained herein. Any reliance on the information presented in this book is at the reader's own risk.

The author and publisher disclaim any liability for any loss, damage, or injury caused or alleged to be caused directly or indirectly by the information contained in this book. It is recommended that readers seek professional advice and guidance where necessary, especially in situations involving mental or physical health.

While every effort has been made to ensure the accuracy and completeness of the information provided, the author and publisher do not assume any responsibility for errors, omissions, or contrary interpretations of the subject matter contained in this book.

The information in this book is subject to change and may be updated or revised at any time without notice.

Defeating Human Papillomavirus (HPV)

The Comprehensive Guide to Prevention, Protection, Treatment, and Management of HPV infection

Henry H. Welch

Table of contents

Introduction

Welcome to the comprehensive guide on Human Papillomavirus (HPV). In the following pages, we will embark on a journey to unravel the mysteries of this common yet often misunderstood viral infection. Our exploration of HPV will encompass various facets, from its basic nature and modes of transmission to the potential health implications it carries and how to protect oneself.

The Importance of Awareness

Understanding HPV is not just a matter of medical knowledge; it is a crucial step towards preventing the adverse effects of this virus. Through this book, we aim to shed light on HPV, its impact on individuals, and the measures that can be taken to manage and, in many cases, prevent it.

As you delve into the chapters that follow, you will gain insights into HPV's prevalence, how it can affect both men and women, and the importance of regular screening. We will discuss testing, treatment options, and preventive measures such as vaccination. Moreover, we will address how HPV can intersect with pregnancy and the potential complications it may pose.

Our journey will be guided by a commitment to providing accurate, up-to-date information about HPV, based on medical research and expert insights. We will navigate this complex subject with clarity and a focus on delivering information that empowers readers to make informed decisions about their health.

Together, we will uncover the truth about Human Papillomavirus, dispelling myths and misconceptions, and equipping you with the knowledge you need to protect yourself and those you care about. Let's embark on this enlightening exploration of HPV, understanding, and awareness.

Chapter 1: What is HPV?

Definition and explanation

Human Papillomavirus (HPV) is a common viral infection that affects the skin and mucous membranes in humans. It is a DNA virus known for its remarkable diversity and its ability to infect various parts of the body, including the genital area, mouth, and throat.

Human Papillomavirus (HPV) is a member of the papillomavirus family, with over 100 different types identified. This highly contagious virus is primarily transmitted through direct skin-to-skin contact. HPV is characterized by its genetic variability, and different types of HPV can be broadly classified into two categories: low-risk and high-risk.

Low-Risk HPV: These HPV types are more likely to cause benign conditions, such as warts (papillomas). While warts can be bothersome, they are generally not associated with cancer.

High-Risk HPV: These are the types of HPV that are more concerning, as they have the potential to lead to more serious health issues, including cancer. Cervical cancer is one of the most well-known cancers associated with high-risk HPV.

Different strains of HPV

Human Papillomavirus (HPV) is not a singular entity but rather a diverse group of viruses, with over 100 distinct types identified. These HPV types can be broadly categorized into two primary groups: low-risk and high-risk strains, each with its own characteristics and implications.

Low-Risk HPV

Low-risk HPV strains are those that are more likely to cause benign conditions and are generally not associated with cancer. However, they can lead to the development of warts, also known as papillomas, in various areas of the body. Some notable low-risk HPV types include:

HPV 6 and 11: These are among the most common low-risk HPV types and are responsible for the majority of genital warts cases.

HPV 1 and 2: These types typically lead to common warts on the hands and fingers.

HPV 3 and 10: These strains can cause flat warts on the face, neck, hands, and wrists.

High-Risk HPV

High-risk HPV strains are the types of HPV that are more concerning due to their potential to lead to more serious health issues, including various cancers. Cervical cancer is one of the most well-recognized cancers associated with high-risk HPV. Some key high-risk HPV types include:

HPV 16 and 18: These are among the most significant high-risk HPV types and are responsible for a substantial portion of cervical cancers. They are also associated with other cancers, such as those of the vulva, vagina, penis, anus, and throat.

HPV 31, 33, 45, 52, and 58: These types are also considered high-risk and can contribute to the development of various cancers.

Understanding the differences between low-risk and high-risk HPV strains is crucial, as it helps to identify the potential health implications associated with each type.

Modes of transmission

Understanding how Human Papillomavirus (HPV) is transmitted is essential to appreciate the full extent of its impact and how it spreads within the population.

Sexual Transmission

HPV is primarily transmitted through direct skin-to-skin contact, making it a sexually transmitted infection (STI). Sexual contact is a key mode of transmission, but it's important to note that intercourse is not the only means by which HPV is spread. Here are the primary sexual transmission methods:

Vaginal Sex: HPV can be transmitted through vaginal sex, even when one partner does not exhibit any symptoms of infection.

Anal Sex: Similar to vaginal sex, anal sex can facilitate the transmission of HPV.

Oral Sex: The virus can also be transmitted through oral-genital contact, leading to HPV infections in the mouth and throat.

Non-Sexual Transmission

While sexual contact is the most common mode of HPV transmission, there are instances of non-sexual transmission as well, including:

Skin-to-Skin Contact: HPV can be transmitted through direct skin-to-skin contact in areas where the virus is present. This contact can lead to the development of warts on the skin.

Vertical Transmission: In rare cases, a mother who carries HPV can transmit the virus to her baby during childbirth. When this occurs, the child may develop a condition known as recurrent respiratory papillomatosis, where HPV-related warts develop inside the child's throat or airways.

Understanding the various modes of HPV transmission highlights the importance of awareness and preventive measures. While HPV is widespread, knowledge about its transmission methods empowers individuals to take steps to protect themselves and prevent the virus from spreading.

Chapter 2: HPV Symptoms and Health Implications

Discuss how HPV often goes unnoticed

Human Papillomavirus (HPV) is a viral infection that often operates stealthily within the human body, going unnoticed by those it infects. This concealment can lead to various implications, including its widespread transmission and potential health risks.

Silent Infection

One of the remarkable aspects of HPV is its ability to cause asymptomatic infections. In fact, the majority of HPV infections do not result in any noticeable symptoms. This means that many individuals can be infected with HPV and remain completely unaware of it.

The silent nature of HPV is attributed to several factors:

Latency Period: HPV infections can have a latency period, during which the virus remains dormant and does not cause any symptoms. This latency period can last for years, making it challenging to detect the virus.

Subclinical Infections: Some HPV infections may be subclinical, meaning they are not associated with visible signs or symptoms. These subclinical infections can persist without causing warts or other noticeable issues.

No Routine Screening: Unlike some other infections, HPV is not routinely screened for in the absence of specific symptoms or risk factors. This lack of routine screening contributes to the silent spread of the virus.

Unaware Transmission

Because many individuals do not experience symptoms and are unaware of their HPV infection, they can unknowingly transmit the virus to their sexual partners. This underlines the significance of HPV education and awareness. Understanding that HPV can exist without symptoms is a crucial step in preventing its spread.

The quiet persistence of HPV in individuals emphasizes the importance of regular check-ups and screenings, as well as the value of vaccination.

Potential health problems caused by HPV

Human Papillomavirus (HPV) is a viral infection that, while often asymptomatic, has the potential to lead to various health problems, especially when the infection does not resolve on its own. We will explore the potential health problems associated with HPV.

Genital Warts

Some HPV infections can lead to the development of **genital warts**, which are growths on or around the genital and anal areas. These warts can be uncomfortable and may cause itching or discomfort. While they are typically benign and not associated with cancer, they can be a source of physical and emotional distress.

Cervical Cancer

Cervical cancer is one of the most well-recognized health problems associated with HPV. High-risk HPV strains, such as HPV 16 and 18, are known to cause changes in cervical cells that can lead to cancer over time. Cervical cancer is a serious and potentially life-threatening condition, highlighting the importance of early detection and prevention.

Other Cancers

In addition to cervical cancer, HPV is linked to various other cancers, including:

Anal Cancer: High-risk HPV types can lead to anal cancer, affecting both men and women. This type of cancer can be challenging to detect and treat.

Penile Cancer: Men can be at risk for penile cancer if they contract high-risk HPV types. Penile cancer is relatively rare but can be serious.

Throat Cancer: High-risk HPV strains, particularly HPV 16, are associated with throat cancer. This type of cancer can affect the base of the tongue and the tonsils.

Warts in the Throat

In rare cases, HPV infections can lead to the development of warts in the throat, a condition known as "recurrent respiratory papillomatosis". This condition can be particularly challenging to manage and can cause respiratory problems.

The potential health problems caused by HPV underscore the importance of awareness, regular screenings, and preventive measures. By understanding the risks and potential consequences associated with HPV, individuals can take steps to protect themselves and seek early medical intervention when necessary.

Chapter 3: HPV in Men

Overview of HPV in men

While Human Papillomavirus (HPV) affects both men and women, its impact on men is a crucial aspect of our exploration.

Prevalence in Men

HPV is highly prevalent in both men and women, and many men may contract the virus during their lifetime. The estimates suggest that up to 80 percent of women and men will contract at least one type of HPV during their lives. However, the prevalence of HPV in men is still significant.

Genital Warts

One of the most common health issues related to HPV in men is the development of genital warts. These warts can appear on the penis, scrotum, and around the anal area. Genital warts can be uncomfortable and may require medical treatment for their removal.

Penile Cancer

High-risk HPV strains, such as HPV 16 and 18, are associated with the development of penile cancer. While penile cancer is relatively rare, HPV remains one of the risk factors for this condition.

Anal Cancer

Men who have sex with men and those with weakened immune systems, such as individuals with HIV, are at a higher risk of developing anal cancer due to HPV infection. High-risk HPV types can lead to anal cancer, making regular screenings and early detection essential.

Throat Cancer

HPV can also affect the throat in men, particularly the base of the tongue and the tonsils. Throat cancer associated with high-risk HPV types, especially HPV 16, is a growing concern and highlights the importance of understanding HPV's impact beyond genital areas.

Importance of Vaccination

Vaccination against HPV is available for both boys and girls. It is a crucial preventive measure to reduce the risk of contracting HPV and the potential health problems it can cause.

Discussion of symptoms and risks

Human Papillomavirus (HPV) is a viral infection known for its ability to remain asymptomatic in many cases. However, when symptoms do occur, they can vary depending on the type of HPV and the specific area of the body affected.

Genital Warts

The most common symptom of HPV, especially low-risk types like HPV 6 and 11, is the development of genital warts. These warts can appear in the genital and anal areas and may cause the following symptoms:

Small, raised growths: Genital warts are typically small, flesh-colored, or gray growths that can be raised or flat.

Itching and discomfort: Genital warts can cause itching or discomfort in the affected areas.

Pain or bleeding during sex: In some cases, genital warts may lead to pain or bleeding during sexual activity.

Respiratory Papillomatosis

In rare cases, especially among infants born to mothers with HPV, the virus can lead to recurrent respiratory papillomatosis, which involves the development of warts in the throat and airways. This condition can lead to respiratory problems and may require surgical intervention.

Risks of HPV

While many HPV infections do not result in noticeable symptoms, the risks associated with the virus are significant, particularly when high-risk HPV types are involved. Some of the key risks of HPV include:

Cervical Cancer

High-risk HPV types, such as HPV 16 and 18, are strongly linked to the development of cervical cancer. This cancer can have serious health consequences and highlights the importance of regular screenings and early detection.

Other Cancers

In addition to cervical cancer, HPV is associated with various other cancers, including:

Anal Cancer: High-risk HPV types can lead to anal cancer, which is more common among men who have sex with men.

Penile Cancer**: Men can be at risk for penile cancer if they contract high-risk HPV types.

Throat Cancer: Throat cancer, particularly in the base of the tongue and tonsils, is associated with high-risk HPV types, primarily HPV 16.

The risks of HPV infections underscore the importance of awareness, preventive measures, and regular screenings. Understanding the potential health consequences of HPV empowers individuals to take proactive steps to protect themselves.

Chapter 4: HPV in Women

Overview of HPV in women

Human Papillomavirus (HPV) is a viral infection that affects both men and women. However, its impact on women is particularly significant due to the specific health risks associated with the virus. We will provide an overview of how HPV can affect women, including the prevalence of the virus and potential health implications.

Prevalence in Women

HPV is highly prevalent among both men and women, with estimates suggesting that up to 80 percent of women and men will contract at least one type of HPV during their lifetime. This high prevalence underscores the importance of understanding HPV's impact on women's health.

Discussion of symptoms and risks

Human Papillomavirus (HPV) can present with various symptoms in women, though it's important to note that many HPV infections are asymptomatic. When symptoms do occur, they can vary depending on the type of HPV and the specific area of the body affected.

Genital Warts

The most common symptom of HPV in women, particularly low-risk types like HPV 6 and 11, is the development of genital warts. These warts can appear in the genital and anal areas and may cause the following symptoms:

Small, raised growths: Genital warts are typically small, flesh-colored, or gray growths that can be raised or flat.

Itching and discomfort: Genital warts can cause itching or discomfort in the affected areas.

Pain or bleeding during sex: In some cases, genital warts may lead to pain or bleeding during sexual activity.

Respiratory Papillomatosis

In rare cases, especially among infants born to mothers with HPV, the virus can lead to recurrent respiratory papillomatosis, which involves the development of warts in the throat and airways. This condition can lead to respiratory problems and may require surgical intervention.

Risks of HPV in Women

While many HPV infections do not result in noticeable symptoms, the risks associated with the virus are significant, especially when high-risk HPV types are involved. Some of the key risks of HPV in women include:

Cervical Cancer

High-risk HPV types, such as HPV 16 and 18, are strongly linked to the development of **cervical cancer**. This cancer can have serious health consequences and highlights the importance of regular screenings and early detection through methods like Pap tests.

Other Cancers

In addition to cervical cancer, HPV is associated with various other types of cancer in women, including:

Vulvar Cancer: High-risk HPV types can lead to the development of vulvar cancer, impacting the external female genitalia.

Vaginal Cancer: HPV is also associated with vaginal cancer, which can have serious health implications.

Throat Cancer: Women can be affected by throat cancer associated with high-risk HPV strains, particularly in the base of the tongue and tonsils.

The symptoms and risks of HPV in women underscore the importance of awareness, preventive measures, and regular screenings. Understanding the potential health consequences of HPV empowers women to take proactive steps to protect themselves and seek early medical intervention when necessary.

Chapter 5: HPV Testing and Screening

Testing guidelines for women

Regular testing and screening for Human Papillomavirus (HPV) are vital for women's health, as the virus is a significant risk factor for various types of cancer, including cervical cancer. In this chapter, I will provide an overview of HPV testing guidelines for women to ensure early detection and effective management.

Pap Smear (Pap Test)

Initial Test: Women should have their first Pap test at age 21, regardless of the onset of sexual activity. The purpose of this initial test is to establish a baseline and begin regular screening.

Ages 21 to 29: Women in this age group should have a Pap test every three years.

Ages 30 to 65: Women in this age range have multiple options for screening:

Pap Test Every Three Years: Women can continue to have a Pap test every three years.

HPV Test Every Five Years: Alternatively, women can choose to have an HPV test every five years. This test screens for high-risk types of HPV (hrHPV).

Co-Testing Every Five Years: Co-testing, which combines a Pap test and an HPV test, can also be done every five years. However, standalone tests are preferred.

Under Age 30: Women younger than age 30 may receive an HPV test if their Pap results are abnormal. This additional testing helps in assessing the presence of high-risk HPV types.

High-Risk HPV Testing

In addition to Pap tests, women may undergo high-risk HPV testing as part of their cervical cancer screening. This test specifically looks for high-risk HPV strains associated with cancer.

It is important to note that women who receive the HPV vaccine should continue with regular cervical cancer screenings, as the vaccine may not protect against all high-risk HPV types.

Follow-Up Testing

If a woman's Pap test or HPV test results are abnormal, follow-up testing and additional screenings may be recommended. This can include procedures such as colposcopy to examine the cervix more closely and potentially remove abnormal or precancerous cells.

By following these testing guidelines, women can take proactive steps to detect and manage HPV-related health issues, particularly cervical cancer. Early detection is crucial in ensuring timely intervention and improving the chances of successful treatment.

Lack of FDA-approved tests for men

While Human Papillomavirus (HPV) affects both men and women, there is a significant disparity in available testing options. Notably, there is a lack of FDA-approved tests specifically designed for diagnosing HPV in men.

HPV DNA Test

The primary test used for HPV diagnosis is the HPV DNA test. This test is widely available and effective for identifying high-risk HPV types in women. However, there is currently no FDA-approved HPV DNA test for diagnosing HPV in men.

Anal Pap Test

Some healthcare providers may perform an anal Pap test for men who are at an increased risk of developing anal cancer due to HPV infection. This is more common in men who have sex with men and individuals with HIV. However, the anal Pap test is not an FDA-approved test for HPV diagnosis.

Lack of Routine Screening

Routine screening for HPV in men, such as the screenings conducted for cervical cancer in women, is not currently recommended by the FDA. This disparity in testing options highlights a gap in healthcare services for men in terms of HPV detection and monitoring.

Importance of Awareness

The lack of FDA-approved tests for men underscores the importance of raising awareness about HPV, its risks, and preventive measures. Men need to be informed about the potential health implications of HPV and the significance of safe sexual practices and vaccination.

Vaccination

While testing options for men are limited, vaccination against HPV is available for boys and men. This preventive measure is crucial in reducing the risk of contracting the virus and the potential health problems it can cause.

By understanding the limitations of HPV testing in men, individuals can take proactive steps to protect themselves and seek early medical intervention when necessary.

Importance of regular screening

Human Papillomavirus (HPV) is a common viral infection with potentially serious health consequences, particularly when it leads to conditions such as cervical cancer and other associated cancers. Regular screening for HPV is of paramount importance for several compelling reasons:

Early Detection

Regular screening, such as Pap tests and HPV DNA tests for women, can lead to the early detection of HPV-related abnormalities in cervical cells. Early detection is critical because it allows for timely medical intervention, increasing the chances of successful treatment and a positive outcome.

Preventing Progression

Detecting HPV-related abnormalities in their early stages can prevent their progression into cancer. Cervical cancer, for instance, often develops slowly, and regular screenings can catch precancerous changes before they become malignant. This makes regular screening an essential tool for preventing cancer.

Improved Survival Rates

For individuals who develop HPV-related cancers, early detection through regular screenings significantly improves survival rates. Cancers detected at later stages are often more challenging to treat and may have lower survival rates.

Peace of Mind

Regular screening provides peace of mind by confirming the absence of HPV-related abnormalities. Knowing that you are in good health can alleviate anxiety and ensure your overall well-being.

Informed Decision-Making

Regular screening empowers individuals to make informed decisions about their health.

If abnormalities are detected, they can work closely with healthcare providers to determine the most appropriate treatment options and create a care plan that best suits their needs.

Prevention Through Vaccination

Regular screenings are essential, but they are not the only defense against HPV-related health issues. HPV vaccination is a crucial preventive measure to protect against the virus and its potential consequences. Combining vaccination with regular screenings provides a comprehensive strategy for managing HPV risks.

Reducing Transmission

Regular screening and vaccination efforts contribute to reducing the transmission of HPV. By preventing infections and catching abnormalities early, the overall prevalence of the virus can be reduced, leading to healthier communities.

In summary, the importance of regular screening for HPV cannot be overstated. It is a fundamental component of maintaining women's health and preventing the development of serious conditions such as cervical cancer.

Follow-up procedures

After an abnormal result from an HPV screening or Pap test, follow-up procedures may be recommended to further evaluate and manage any detected abnormalities. These procedures are essential in ensuring that potential health issues are addressed promptly and appropriately. Here, we will discuss common follow-up procedures for HPV abnormalities.

Colposcopy

A "colposcopy" is a procedure in which a healthcare provider uses a special magnifying instrument called a colposcope to closely examine the cervix, vagina, and vulva. This procedure is often recommended when an abnormality is detected in a Pap test or when high-risk HPV is present.

During a colposcopy, the healthcare provider can:

- Identify abnormal areas on the cervix.
- Take tissue samples (biopsies) from suspicious areas for further evaluation.
- Assess the severity of the abnormality and its potential to progress to cancer.

Biopsy

A "biopsy" is the removal of a small sample of tissue for laboratory analysis. This is typically done during a colposcopy when abnormal areas are identified. Biopsies help determine the nature and extent of abnormalities and whether further treatment is required.

There are different types of biopsies, including:

- **Cervical Biopsy:** A sample of tissue is taken from the cervix.
- **Endocervical Curettage:** Cells are scraped from the cervical canal.
- **Loop Electrosurgical Excision Procedure (LEEP):** A thin wire loop with an electrical current is used to remove abnormal tissue.

Additional Testing

Depending on the results of a colposcopy and biopsy, additional testing and diagnostic procedures may be necessary. These may include:

- **Imaging:** In some cases, imaging studies such as magnetic resonance imaging (MRI) or computed tomography (CT) scans may be conducted to assess the extent of the abnormality.

- **Treatment Planning:** After a thorough evaluation, a healthcare provider will determine the most appropriate treatment plan, which may include surgery, cryotherapy, or other interventions.

Regular Monitoring

For some individuals, follow-up procedures may involve regular monitoring and surveillance to track the progression or regression of HPV-related abnormalities. In many cases, low-grade abnormalities may resolve on their own without the need for invasive treatment.

It's essential to follow healthcare provider recommendations for follow-up procedures, as they are designed to catch potential issues at an early stage and ensure timely intervention when needed. These procedures are crucial in managing HPV-related health concerns and preventing the development of cancer. In the upcoming chapters, we will delve into available treatment options and discuss the significance of vaccination in further detail, equipping you with the knowledge needed to manage HPV-related health risks effectively.

Chapter 6: HPV Treatment and Management

The natural course of HPV infections

Understanding the natural course of Human Papillomavirus (HPV) infections is crucial in comprehending how the virus can affect individuals over time. HPV infections can follow various paths, and their outcomes depend on factors such as the type of HPV, the individual's immune response, and other contributing factors. In this chapter, we will explore the natural course of HPV infections.

Self-Resolution

A significant proportion of HPV infections undergo self-resolution. This means that the body's immune system can clear the virus naturally over time. In fact, approximately 90 percent of HPV infections resolve on their own within two years, according to the Centers for Disease Control and Prevention (CDC). Self-resolution often occurs without any noticeable symptoms or health problems.

Persistent Infection

In some cases, HPV infections do not resolve on their own and become persistent. This persistence can lead to various health issues, including the development of genital warts and, in the case of high-risk HPV types, the progression to cancer.

Genital Warts

Low-risk HPV types, such as HPV 6 and 11, are responsible for the development of genital warts. When the virus persists, it can cause warts to appear in the genital and anal areas. These warts can be uncomfortable and may require medical treatment for their removal.

Cancer Risk

High-risk HPV types, particularly HPV 16 and 18, are strongly associated with the development of cancer. Persistent infection with high-risk HPV strains can lead to changes in cervical cells, which may progress to cervical cancer over time. This highlights the critical importance of regular screenings and early detection to monitor and manage HPV-related abnormalities.

Watchful Waiting

For individuals with low-grade HPV-related abnormalities, healthcare providers may recommend a course of watchful waiting. This approach involves monitoring the situation and conducting regular screenings to assess whether the abnormalities progress or regress over time. It is an option for cases where immediate intervention is not necessary.

Importance of Regular Screenings

Regular screenings, such as Pap tests and HPV tests, are essential in identifying and monitoring HPV-related abnormalities. These screenings can detect changes in cervical cells early, enabling timely intervention and improving the chances of successful treatment. By understanding the natural course of HPV infections, individuals can make informed decisions about their healthcare and take proactive steps to protect themselves.

Treatment of genital warts

Genital warts, which are caused by certain strains of Human Papillomavirus (HPV), can be uncomfortable and concerning. Fortunately, various treatment options are available to manage and remove these warts. In this chapter, we will explore the treatments for genital warts.

Topical Treatments

Podofilox (Condylox): A topical solution that can be applied to the warts. It is generally applied twice a day for three days, followed by four days of no treatment. This cycle can be repeated as needed.

Imiquimod (Aldara, Zyclara): A topical cream that stimulates the body's immune system to fight the virus. It is typically applied before bedtime and washed off in the morning, three times a week.

Sinecatechins (Veregen): An ointment that can be applied three times daily to external genital and perianal warts.

In-Office Procedures

Cryotherapy (Cryosurgery): In this procedure, a healthcare provider uses liquid nitrogen to freeze and remove warts. It may require several sessions.

Electrocautery: This method involves burning off warts using an electrical current.

Surgical Excision: In some cases, the healthcare provider may surgically remove warts. This is typically recommended for large warts or those that have not responded to other treatments.

Interferon Injections

Injections of interferon, a medication that can boost the immune system's response, may be used for persistent or recurrent genital warts. These injections are typically administered by a healthcare provider.

Laser Therapy

In certain cases, laser therapy may be used to remove genital warts. This method uses a laser to target and vaporize the warts.

Self-Applied Treatments

Trichloroacetic Acid (TCA): TCA is a chemical compound that can be applied by the individual directly to the warts. It works by causing the cells of the warts to break down.

It is important to note that while treatments can remove visible warts, they do not cure the underlying HPV infection. HPV can persist in the body even after warts are removed, which is why regular screenings and follow-up care are crucial.

Preventing Transmission

During treatment and recovery, it is essential to practice safe sex to prevent the transmission of HPV to sexual partners. Condoms can provide some level of protection but are not foolproof, as HPV can infect areas not covered by a condom.

Follow-Up

After treatment, individuals should closely follow their healthcare provider's recommendations for follow-up appointments and screenings to monitor for recurrence and potential complications.

The treatment of genital warts is a multi-faceted approach that can involve various methods, depending on the size, location, and number of warts. It is crucial to consult with a healthcare provider to determine the most appropriate treatment plan for individual cases.

Addressing precancerous cells

When the Human Papillomavirus (HPV) infection leads to the development of precancerous cells, timely intervention is essential to prevent the progression to cancer. In this chapter, we will explore the methods and procedures used to address precancerous cells caused by HPV.

Colposcopy and Biopsy

The first step in addressing precancerous cells is often a **colposcopy**. During this procedure, a healthcare provider uses a colposcope to closely examine the cervix, vagina, and vulva. If abnormal areas are identified, a "biopsy" may be performed to collect tissue samples for further evaluation.

Diagnostic Procedures

In cases of precancerous cells, the following diagnostic procedures may be recommended:

Cervical Biopsy: A sample of tissue is taken from the cervix to determine the extent of abnormality.

Endocervical Curettage: Cells from the cervical canal are scraped and collected for analysis.

Loop Electrosurgical Excision Procedure (LEEP): Abnormal tissue can be removed using a thin wire loop with an electrical current.

Assessing Severity

The results of these diagnostic procedures help determine the severity of the precancerous cells. Precancerous cells are typically classified into different categories, including:

Cervical Intraepithelial Neoplasia (CIN) I, II, and III: These categories represent the degree of abnormality, with CIN III being the most severe.

Atypical Squamous Cells of Undetermined Significance (ASCUS): This indicates that the changes in cervical cells are unclear and require further evaluation.

Treatment Options

The appropriate treatment for precancerous cells depends on their severity and location. Common treatment options include:

- **Cryotherapy (Cryosurgery):** Freezing abnormal cells to destroy them.

- **Laser Therapy:** Using a laser to vaporize abnormal tissue.
- **Cone Biopsy (Conization):** Removing a cone-shaped piece of tissue from the cervix.

- **Hysterectomy:** In severe cases, the removal of the uterus may be recommended.

Regular Monitoring

After treatment, individuals with a history of precancerous cells are typically placed on a regular monitoring schedule. This includes follow-up screenings and colposcopies to ensure that any recurrence or progression is detected and addressed promptly.

It is essential to follow healthcare provider recommendations closely and maintain a consistent schedule of screenings and follow-up appointments to effectively manage precancerous cells caused by HPV. Timely intervention and regular monitoring are key to preventing the development of cancer.

Treatment of HPV-related cancers

When Human Papillomavirus (HPV) infections lead to the development of cancers, it becomes crucial to pursue appropriate treatment strategies.

HPV-related cancers, such as cervical cancer, anal cancer, and oropharyngeal cancer, require specialized care.

Cervical Cancer

Surgery: Depending on the stage of cervical cancer, surgical options may include the removal of cancerous tissue, the uterus (hysterectomy), or lymph nodes. In some cases, a radical trachelectomy, which removes the cervix but preserves fertility, may be an option.

Radiation Therapy: High-energy X-rays are used to target and destroy cancer cells. This may be used in combination with surgery or chemotherapy.

Chemotherapy: Medications are administered to kill cancer cells or slow their growth. Chemotherapy may be used alone or in combination with surgery and radiation therapy.

Targeted Therapy: This treatment targets specific molecules involved in cancer growth and may be used in conjunction with chemotherapy.

Immunotherapy: Immunotherapy harnesses the body's immune system to fight cancer cells. It is an evolving field of cancer treatment and may be utilized in certain cases.

Anal Cancer

Surgery: Surgical options for anal cancer include removing the cancerous tissue or the entire anal canal (abdominoperineal resection).

Chemoradiation: A combination of chemotherapy and radiation therapy is often the primary treatment for anal cancer.

Targeted Therapy: Similar to cervical cancer, targeted therapy may be utilized in some cases.

Oropharyngeal Cancer

Surgery: Depending on the extent of oropharyngeal cancer, surgery may involve removing the tumor or a portion of the affected tissue.

Radiation Therapy: Radiation therapy is commonly used to treat oropharyngeal cancer, either alone or in combination with surgery.

Chemotherapy: Chemotherapy may be administered alongside radiation therapy or surgery.

Immunotherapy: Emerging as a promising treatment option, immunotherapy is being studied for its effectiveness in treating oropharyngeal cancer.

Multidisciplinary Approach

HPV-related cancer treatment often involves a multidisciplinary approach. A team of healthcare providers, including oncologists, surgeons, radiation therapists, and other specialists, collaborate to create a tailored treatment plan based on the specific cancer type and stage.

Survivorship Care

After cancer treatment, survivorship care becomes essential. This includes regular follow-up appointments, screenings, and support to manage potential side effects of treatment.

Prevention and Early Detection

While treatment options for HPV-related cancers have advanced significantly, prevention and early detection remain fundamental. HPV vaccination and regular screenings are critical in reducing the incidence of these cancers and improving treatment outcomes.

Ongoing Research

Ongoing research continues to explore new and innovative approaches to treating HPV-related cancers. Clinical trials may offer opportunities for individuals with these cancers to access cutting-edge treatments.

It is important to consult with healthcare providers who specialize in cancer care to determine the most appropriate treatment plan for HPV-related cancers. By understanding the available treatment options and the importance of prevention, individuals can make informed decisions about their healthcare.

Chapter 7: HPV Prevention

Safe sex practices

Practicing safe sex is essential not only for preventing Human Papillomavirus (HPV) but also for reducing the risk of other sexually transmitted infections (STIs). HPV can be transmitted through intimate sexual contact, but there are steps individuals can take to protect themselves and their partners.

Condom Use

Latex or Polyurethane Condoms: Consistently and correctly using latex or polyurethane condoms during sexual activity can significantly reduce the risk of HPV transmission. Condoms create a barrier that can help prevent the exchange of bodily fluids and skin contact.

Dental Dams

Dental Dams: For oral sex, dental dams can be used to create a barrier between the mouth and the genital area. This can help reduce the risk of oral HPV transmission.

Vaccination

HPV Vaccination: One of the most effective ways to prevent HPV infection is through vaccination. The HPV vaccine is available for both males and females, and it provides protection against the most common high-risk HPV types. Vaccination is recommended for adolescents and young adults, but it can be administered up to age 45 for those who haven't previously been vaccinated.

Limiting Sexual Partners

Monogamy: Reducing the number of sexual partners and being in a mutually monogamous relationship can lower the risk of HPV transmission.

Regular Screenings

Regular Screenings: For those at risk of HPV-related cancers, such as cervical cancer, regular screenings are essential. Early detection can lead to timely intervention and improved treatment outcomes.

Education and Communication

Education and Communication: Open and honest communication with sexual partners is key to making informed decisions about sexual health. Individuals should discuss their sexual history and STI testing.

Abstinence

Abstinence: The only surefire way to avoid HPV and other STIs is abstinence from sexual activity.

It is important to note that while these safe sex practices can reduce the risk of HPV transmission, they do not eliminate it entirely. HPV can infect areas not covered by condoms, and the virus can persist even after the visible warts have been removed. Therefore, a combination of safe sex practices and vaccination is the most effective approach to preventing HPV and its associated health risks.

Gardasil 9 vaccine

One of the most significant breakthroughs in preventing Human Papillomavirus (HPV) infections, including the most common high-risk types, is the development of the Gardasil 9 vaccine. This vaccine has revolutionized HPV prevention, offering protection against a broad range of HPV strains.

What is Gardasil 9?

Gardasil 9 is a vaccine designed to provide protection against nine different types of HPV, including the most common high-risk types (HPV 16 and 18) and the types responsible for genital warts (HPV 6 and 11). It is a follow-up to the original Gardasil vaccine, which protected against four HPV types.

Types of HPV Covered

Gardasil 9 targets the following HPV types:

HPV 16 and 18: Responsible for most HPV-related cancers, including cervical, anal, and oropharyngeal cancers.

HPV 6 and 11: The main culprits behind genital warts.

HPV 31, 33, 45, 52, and 58: Additional high-risk types linked to cervical and other cancers.

Who Should Get Vaccinated?

Gardasil 9 is recommended for both males and females. The vaccine is most effective when administered before exposure to HPV through sexual activity. As a result, it is typically recommended for adolescents and young adults. In the United States, the Centers for Disease Control and Prevention (CDC) recommends routine vaccination at age 11 or 12.

Gardasil 9 can also be administered to individuals up to age 45 who haven't previously been vaccinated, although the vaccine's effectiveness may decrease with age.

Dosing Schedule

The vaccine is administered in a series of shots. The dosing schedule typically involves two or three doses, depending on the individual's age at the time of the first dose.

Effectiveness

Gardasil 9 is highly effective at preventing the HPV types it targets. It has significantly reduced the prevalence of these HPV strains in populations where vaccination rates are high. As a result, it has the potential to reduce the incidence of HPV-related cancers and genital warts.

Safety

The vaccine has undergone extensive testing and is considered safe. Like any vaccine, it may cause mild side effects such as pain at the injection site, fever, or dizziness. Serious side effects are extremely rare.

Importance of Vaccination

The Gardasil 9 vaccine plays a crucial role in reducing the burden of HPV-related diseases, including cancer. By getting vaccinated, individuals not only protect themselves but also contribute to the establishment of herd immunity, which benefits the broader community by reducing the circulation of HPV.

Recommendations for vaccination

Vaccination against Human Papillomavirus (HPV) is a critical public health measure to reduce the prevalence of HPV-related diseases, including various cancers and genital warts.

Routine Vaccination

The Centers for Disease Control and Prevention (CDC) and other health organizations recommend routine HPV vaccination for the following groups:

Adolescents and Young Adults: The primary target group for routine HPV vaccination is adolescents and young adults. The CDC recommends vaccination for:

- All children at age 11 or 12. Vaccination at this age is highly effective, as it is before potential exposure to HPV through sexual activity.

- Teens and young adults through age 26 who have not been previously vaccinated.

Catch-Up Vaccination: For individuals who were not vaccinated during adolescence, catch-up vaccination is recommended for:

- Females through age 26.

- Males through age 21.

Shared Decision-Making: The CDC suggests shared decision-making for adults aged 27 to 45 who have not been vaccinated. While vaccination may still provide some benefits, its effectiveness tends to decrease with age. Therefore, individuals in this age group should discuss the pros and cons of vaccination with their healthcare providers.

Multiple Doses

HPV vaccination is typically administered as a series of shots. The number of doses required depends on the individual's age at the time of the first dose:

Age 11 or 12: Two doses, given six to twelve months apart.

Aged 15 or older: Three doses, with the second dose administered one to two months after the first, and the third dose six months after the first.

Importance of Completion

It is essential to complete the recommended number of doses for the vaccine to be most effective. Incomplete vaccination may not provide the same level of protection against HPV.

Herd Immunity

High vaccination rates not only protect individuals but also contribute to herd immunity. Herd immunity occurs when a significant portion of the population is immune to a disease, reducing its spread. This helps protect those who cannot be vaccinated, such as individuals with certain medical conditions.

Safe and Effective

The HPV vaccine, including Gardasil 9, is safe and highly effective at preventing the targeted HPV types. It has been extensively tested and is considered a critical tool in reducing the burden of HPV-related diseases.

Parental Consent

In most cases, parental or guardian consent is required for minors to receive the HPV vaccine. It is important for parents and guardians to stay informed about the vaccine's benefits and to discuss vaccination with healthcare providers.

Importance of regular checkups and screenings

Regular checkups and screenings play a crucial role in managing Human Papillomavirus (HPV) infections and preventing the development of associated health problems. In this chapter, we will explore why consistent healthcare monitoring is essential for individuals at risk of HPV.

Early Detection

One of the primary benefits of regular checkups and screenings is **early detection**. HPV infections, especially high-risk types, can lead to the development of precancerous or cancerous changes in the cervix, anus, or oropharynx. Early detection through screenings allows for timely intervention and treatment, significantly improving treatment outcomes.

Cervical Cancer Screening

For individuals with cervixes, regular cervical cancer screenings are critical. These screenings can detect changes in cervical cells caused by HPV, known as cervical intraepithelial neoplasia (CIN). Early detection of CIN allows for the removal of precancerous cells before they progress to cancer.

-**Pap Tests:** A Pap test, also known as a Pap smear, is used to collect cells from the cervix for analysis. It can identify abnormal changes that may require further evaluation.

- **HPV Tests:** In addition to Pap tests, HPV tests can identify the presence of high-risk HPV types that are linked to cervical cancer. Co-testing with Pap and HPV tests is a recommended approach for women aged 30 to 65.

Anal Cancer Screening

For individuals at risk of anal cancer, including men who have sex with men (MSM), regular anal Pap tests may be recommended. These tests can detect precancerous changes in anal cells.

Oropharyngeal Cancer Screening

Oropharyngeal cancer, often linked to HPV, may require regular screenings for individuals at risk, including those with a history of smoking or heavy alcohol use. Screenings involve visual and physical examinations by healthcare providers.

Vaccination and Screenings

Vaccination against HPV is highly effective in preventing the most common high-risk types. However, even vaccinated individuals should continue with regular screenings as the vaccine does not provide protection against all high-risk types.

Follow-Up Care

When screenings detect abnormal changes, follow-up care and interventions are crucial. This may involve additional testing, colposcopy, biopsies, and treatment procedures to address precancerous or cancerous cells.

Personalized Care

Healthcare providers can offer personalized guidance on the appropriate timing and frequency of screenings based on individual risk factors, including sexual activity, vaccination status, and medical history.

Peace of Mind

Regular checkups and screenings provide individuals with peace of mind, knowing that they are taking proactive steps to monitor their health and detect any issues early. This reduces anxiety and uncertainty related to potential HPV-related health problems.

Public Health Impact

By participating in regular screenings and follow-up care, individuals contribute to the broader **public health impact** of reducing the prevalence of HPV-related diseases. This not only benefits their own health but also the health of their communities.

Chapter 8: HPV and Pregnancy

How HPV affects pregnancy

Human Papillomavirus (HPV) can impact various aspects of pregnancy, from conception to childbirth. In this chapter, we will explore how HPV may affect pregnancy, potential complications, and important considerations for expectant parents.

HPV and Fertility

Fertility Impact: HPV typically does not affect fertility. However, in some cases, extensive genital warts might cause blockages or obstructions in the reproductive organs, potentially impacting fertility.

HPV Treatment and Fertility: Treatments for genital warts, such as cryotherapy or laser therapy, aim to remove warts while preserving fertility. It's important for healthcare providers to discuss potential effects on fertility with patients before treatment.

HPV and Pregnancy

Transmission to the Baby: While it's rare, there is a risk of HPV transmission from the mother to the baby during childbirth. This can lead to a condition known as **recurrent respiratory papillomatosis (RRP)**, where warts develop in the baby's throat or airways.

Caesarean Section: In cases where the mother has visible genital warts, a

healthcare provider may recommend a
caesarean section (C-section) to reduce
the risk of HPV transmission to the baby.
The decision to perform a C-section is made
on a case-by-case basis.

Pap Smears During Pregnancy

Continuing Pap Smears: Pregnant
individuals should continue to have regular
Pap smears during pregnancy. Early
detection and management of any cervical
changes related to HPV are essential.

Hormonal Changes

Genital Warts During Pregnancy:
Some pregnant individuals may experience
changes in their genital warts due to
hormonal fluctuations during pregnancy.
This may include warts growing in size or
bleeding.

Postpartum Changes: In some cases, genital warts may resolve on their own postpartum, while in others, they may persist and require treatment.

Vaccination During Pregnancy

Vaccination Timing: The HPV vaccine is not recommended during pregnancy. Therefore, it is advisable for individuals to consider vaccination before becoming pregnant.

Shared Decision-Making

Discussing HPV and Pregnancy: Pregnant individuals with HPV should have open discussions with their healthcare providers to address any concerns or questions. Healthcare providers can provide guidance on how to manage HPV-related issues during pregnancy.

Counseling: Genetic counseling may be recommended for individuals with HPV who are planning a family. This can help address any concerns related to HPV and pregnancy.

HPV Vaccination for Children

Protecting Future Generations: One of the best ways to protect future generations from HPV-related complications during pregnancy is to ensure children receive the HPV vaccine according to recommended schedules.

Emotional Support

Emotional Impact: The emotional impact of dealing with HPV during pregnancy can be significant. Seek emotional support from healthcare providers, counselors, or support groups when needed.

Delaying treatment during pregnancy

Pregnancy can bring about unique considerations when it comes to managing Human Papillomavirus (HPV) and related conditions. In this chapter, we will explore the circumstances in which treatment for HPV may be delayed during pregnancy and the reasons behind these decisions.

Treatment Timing

Consideration of Treatment: For individuals with HPV-related conditions such as genital warts or abnormal cervical cells, the timing of treatment during pregnancy is a decision made in consultation with healthcare providers.

Delaying Treatment

Genital Warts: In some cases, healthcare providers may recommend delaying treatment for genital warts during pregnancy. This is often because the warts may resolve on their own postpartum, and treatment can be postponed to avoid potential harm to the developing fetus.

Cervical Procedures: Delaying treatments like colposcopy or cervical biopsies during pregnancy is common practice. These procedures involve taking tissue samples from the cervix, and while they are generally safe, they may be deferred to avoid potential risks.

Cervical Changes and Follow-Up

Cervical Changes: Regular follow-up through Pap tests and HPV testing is essential for pregnant individuals with known cervical changes. This allows healthcare providers to monitor any progression of these changes and make informed decisions about postpartum treatment.

Warts and Childbirth

Visible Genital Warts: If visible genital warts are present during childbirth, healthcare providers may recommend a caesarean section to reduce the risk of transmission to the baby.

Case-by-Case Decisions: The decision to perform a C-section is made on a case-by-case basis, taking into account the size and location of the warts.

Emotional Support

Emotional Impact: Dealing with HPV-related conditions and treatment decisions during pregnancy can be emotionally challenging. Seeking emotional support from healthcare providers, counselors, or support groups is valuable.

Future Planning

Postpartum Care: Postpartum care may involve resuming or starting HPV-related treatments or interventions that were delayed during pregnancy.

Vaccination: Consideration of the HPV vaccine after pregnancy is an option for those who haven't been vaccinated. Healthcare providers can provide guidance on vaccination timing.

Family Planning: For individuals who wish to have more children, future family planning should involve discussions with healthcare providers to address HPV-related concerns.

Complications and C-section

In pregnancies where Human Papillomavirus (HPV) is present, certain complications may arise, potentially leading to the recommendation of a caesarean section (C-section) for the safety of both the mother and the baby. This chapter delves into the complications that may warrant a C-section in HPV-related pregnancies.

Visible Genital Warts

Risk of Transmission: When visible genital warts are present during childbirth, there is a risk of transmitting HPV to the baby. This risk primarily stems from contact with the warts.

Risk to the Baby: The transmission of HPV to the baby can result in recurrent respiratory papillomatosis (RRP), a rare condition where warts develop in the baby's throat or airways.

Consideration for C-Section: In cases of visible genital warts, healthcare providers may recommend a caesarean section to minimize the risk of HPV transmission to the baby.

Case-by-Case Decision: The decision to perform a C-section is individualized and made based on factors such as the size and location of the warts and the potential risk to the baby.

C-Section and Maternal Health

Maternal Health: A caesarean section, while ensuring the baby's safety in the presence of visible genital warts, also serves to protect the mother's health by reducing the risk of tearing or damage to the genital warts during vaginal childbirth.

Preserving Fertility: C-sections aim to minimize the risk of damaging the genital warts, preserving fertility, and reducing potential complications during and after childbirth.

Preparing for C-Section

Communication: Pregnant individuals with HPV-related complications should have open and honest discussions with their healthcare providers about the possibility of a C-section and any associated risks.

Timing: The timing of a C-section may be planned in advance or scheduled as needed, often close to the due date.

Healthcare Team: The healthcare team, including obstetricians and infectious disease specialists, works together to ensure a safe and successful C-section.

Postpartum Care: After a C-section, postpartum care and follow-up are crucial, including monitoring the healing process and addressing any residual HPV-related conditions.

Emotional Support

Emotional Impact: Dealing with the possibility of a C-section due to HPV-related complications can be emotionally challenging. Emotional support is valuable, and individuals should seek guidance from healthcare providers, counselors, or support groups.

Recurrent respiratory papillomatosis

Recurrent Respiratory Papillomatosis (RRP) is a rare but potentially serious condition caused by the Human Papillomavirus (HPV).

What is RRP?

RRP is a condition characterized by the growth of warts or papillomas in the respiratory tract. These growths can occur in the larynx (voice box), trachea (windpipe), and other parts of the respiratory system.

Causes

HPV-Related: RRP is primarily caused by HPV, specifically high-risk types such as

HPV 6 and 11. These types are also associated with genital warts.

Transmission to Infants: In some cases, infants born to mothers with genital warts caused by these high-risk HPV types can develop RRP. This occurs when the baby is exposed to the virus during childbirth.

Symptoms

Respiratory Symptoms: The most common symptoms of RRP are related to the respiratory system. These may include hoarseness, difficulty breathing, chronic cough, and noisy breathing.

Severity Varies: The severity of RRP can vary widely among individuals. Some may have only a few growths that cause mild symptoms, while others may experience more extensive growths leading to severe breathing difficulties.

Diagnosis

Laryngoscopy: Diagnosis of RRP typically involves a laryngoscopy, where a flexible tube with a camera is inserted through the nose or mouth to visualize the larynx and other areas of the respiratory tract.

Biopsy: In some cases, a biopsy may be taken to confirm the presence of papillomas and identify the HPV type responsible.

Treatment

Management: The primary treatment for RRP is the removal of papillomas. This is typically done through minimally invasive procedures, such as laser therapy or microdebriders, which help minimize damage to surrounding tissue.

Frequency: The recurrence of papillomas is common in RRP, and repeated procedures may be necessary.

Vocal Cord Care: For individuals with vocal cord involvement, voice therapy and careful management of vocal cord health are essential.

HPV Vaccination: The HPV vaccine can provide protection against the HPV types most commonly associated with RRP, offering a preventive measure for both children and adults.

Emotional Impact

Emotional Challenges: Dealing with RRP can be emotionally challenging, particularly for children and parents. Emotional support and counseling may be beneficial in managing the impact of the condition.

Ongoing Monitoring

Regular Follow-Up: Individuals with RRP require ongoing monitoring and follow-up care to assess the status of papillomas and ensure timely treatment when necessary.

Chapter 9: HPV Facts and Statistics

Prevalence of HPV in the United States

Human Papillomavirus (HPV) is a common sexually transmitted infection with a significant impact on public health.

Prevalence Statistics

Highly Prevalent: HPV is one of the most prevalent sexually transmitted infections in the United States. It is estimated that approximately 79 million Americans are currently infected with HPV.

Common Infection: The majority of sexually active individuals will contract at least one type of HPV during their lifetime, often shortly after becoming sexually active.

Age Groups: HPV prevalence is highest among young adults and adolescents, with the peak occurring in individuals aged 20 to 24.

Gender Disparities

Gender Differences: The prevalence of HPV varies between genders. Research indicates that men are slightly more likely to be infected with high-risk HPV types than women.

Impact on Men: High-risk HPV types in men can lead to conditions such as penile, anal, and throat cancers.

Impact on Women: For women, HPV can result in cervical cancer and other genital cancers.

Racial and Ethnic Disparities

Disparities: There are racial and ethnic disparities in HPV prevalence. Some communities may have higher rates of infection.

Access to Healthcare: These disparities can be influenced by factors such as access to healthcare, vaccination rates, and sexual behavior.

Vaccination Impact

Impact of Vaccination: The introduction of HPV vaccines, such as Gardasil 9, has had a positive impact on reducing the prevalence of high-risk HPV types. Vaccination is recommended for both boys and girls to prevent HPV-related health problems.

Public Health Initiatives

Prevention Strategies: Public health initiatives in the United States emphasize the importance of HPV vaccination, early detection through screenings, and safe sex practices.

Screening Programs: Regular Pap tests and HPV testing for women, as well as anal Pap tests for some men, are part of screening programs designed to identify and manage HPV-related conditions.

Education: Education campaigns aim to increase awareness about the risks of HPV and the benefits of vaccination, especially among adolescents and young adults.

Ongoing Research

Research Efforts: Ongoing research is focused on understanding HPV prevalence, identifying trends, and developing effective prevention and treatment strategies.

Annual contraction rates

Human Papillomavirus (HPV) is a dynamic infection with varying annual contraction rates that reflect the changing landscape of HPV prevalence and its impact on public health.

Fluctuating Annual Rates

Dynamic Infection: HPV is a dynamic infection with fluctuating annual contraction rates. These rates can change based on several factors, including vaccination campaigns and sexual behavior.

Vaccination Impact

Vaccination Campaigns: The introduction of HPV vaccines, such as Gardasil 9, has had a notable impact on reducing the contraction of certain high-risk HPV types. The success of vaccination campaigns contributes to lower annual contraction rates.

Vaccination Coverage: The effectiveness of vaccination in reducing annual contraction rates is influenced by the coverage and uptake of the vaccine, especially among adolescents and young adults.

Sexual Behavior

Key Influence: Sexual behavior plays a significant role in determining annual contraction rates. Factors such as the number of sexual partners, sexual activity, and use of protection can influence the likelihood of contracting HPV.

Safer Sex Practices: Practicing safe sex, including consistent condom use and limiting the number of sexual partners, can help reduce the risk of contracting HPV.

Age and Demographics

Age Groups: HPV contraction rates can vary among different age groups. Adolescents and young adults are often at a higher risk of contracting HPV due to sexual debut and sexual activity.

Demographic Differences: HPV contraction rates can also differ by demographic factors, including race, ethnicity, and socioeconomic status.

Screening and Detection

Screening Programs: The availability and effectiveness of screening programs, such as Pap tests and HPV testing, can impact the detection of HPV and influence contraction rates.

Early Detection: Early detection through screenings can help identify HPV-related conditions and initiate timely treatment.

Public Health Initiatives

Preventive Measures: Public health initiatives, education campaigns, and the promotion of HPV vaccination are essential in reducing annual contraction rates and preventing HPV-related health problems.

Awareness: Raising awareness about the risks of HPV and the importance of vaccination is a key component of public health efforts.

Ongoing Surveillance

Research and Surveillance: Ongoing research and surveillance efforts monitor annual contraction rates, track trends, and inform public health policies and strategies.

Impact of vaccination

The introduction of Human Papillomavirus (HPV) vaccines has had a significant impact on public health by reducing the prevalence of HPV infection and related health problems. In this chapter, we will explore the substantial impact of HPV vaccination on preventing HPV-related diseases.

Reduction in Prevalence

Lower HPV Rates: HPV vaccination has resulted in a reduction in the prevalence of high-risk HPV types, particularly HPV 16 and 18, which are associated with various cancers.

Herd Immunity: High vaccination rates in a population create herd immunity, protecting even those who are unvaccinated by reducing the overall transmission of the virus.

Cervical Cancer Prevention

Cervical Cancer: HPV vaccination significantly lowers the risk of cervical cancer, as it targets the types most commonly responsible for this cancer.

Preventing Precancerous Changes: By preventing high-risk HPV infections, vaccination also reduces the occurrence of precancerous changes in the cervix.

Impact on Other Cancers

Other Cancers: HPV vaccination has the potential to reduce the risk of other cancers, including those of the vulva, vagina, anus, and oropharynx (back of the throat).

Anal Cancer: In men, vaccination can help prevent anal cancer, particularly in those who have sex with men.

Genital Warts Reduction

Genital Warts: HPV vaccines have been effective in reducing the incidence of genital warts, providing relief to those affected by this common HPV-related condition.

Vaccination Timing

Early Vaccination: HPV vaccination is most effective when administered at a young age, ideally before the onset of sexual activity.

Adolescents and Young Adults: Routine vaccination is recommended for both boys and girls aged 11 or 12, with catch-up vaccination available for those up to age 26.

Future Impact

Continued Reduction: As more individuals receive the HPV vaccine, the impact on reducing HPV-related diseases is expected to grow.

Research and Development: Ongoing research and the development of new HPV vaccines may further enhance prevention efforts.

Public Health Initiatives

Promotion of Vaccination: Public health campaigns emphasize the importance of HPV vaccination for adolescents and young adults, promoting awareness and vaccine uptake.

Education: Education efforts inform individuals and parents about the benefits of vaccination and dispel myths and concerns.

Global Impact

Global Efforts: HPV vaccination is a critical component of global public health initiatives to reduce the burden of HPV-related diseases worldwide.

Conclusion

The Human Papillomavirus (HPV) is a widespread infection with a profound impact on public health. In this comprehensive exploration of HPV, we have uncovered the various aspects of this virus, from its prevalence and transmission to its association with diseases and the transformative effects of vaccination.

We have delved into the depths of HPV, understanding that it is a virus of many facets, some of which may go unnoticed, posing challenges for early detection and prevention. We have explored how HPV often eludes detection, silently residing in the body, with most infections resolving spontaneously but some leading to severe health problems.

Throughout this journey, we have navigated the gender-specific impacts of HPV, from genital warts and cancers in men to cervical, vaginal, and vulvar cancers in women. We have highlighted the significance of regular screenings for both genders and discussed the limitations in HPV testing for men, shedding light on the need for continued research and development in this area.

We have acknowledged the importance of vaccination in the fight against HPV, with the advent of vaccines like Gardasil 9 that have already made a remarkable difference in reducing the prevalence of high-risk HPV types and the associated cancers. The impact of vaccination extends to the prevention of other cancers and the reduction of genital warts, ushering in a new era of public health.

As we conclude this comprehensive journey through the world of HPV, we emphasize the need for continued research, public health initiatives, education, and awareness campaigns. By empowering individuals with knowledge, encouraging vaccination, and promoting safe sex practices, we can collectively work toward a future where HPV-related diseases are rarer and less severe.

HPV is a formidable adversary, but with the right tools and strategies, we can stand strong in the fight against this invisible yet potent virus. Our hope is that the knowledge gained from this exploration serves as a foundation for a healthier future, free from the burdens of HPV-related diseases.

Thank you for embarking on this journey through the complex and multifaceted world of HPV. Your understanding, awareness, and commitment to prevention make a meaningful difference in the battle against this pervasive virus.

In the realm of public health, knowledge is a powerful weapon, and together, we can continue to wield it to protect future generations from the impact of HPV.